RISING

Jackie Ng

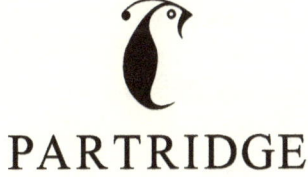

PARTRIDGE

To order additional copies of this book, contact
Toll Free +65 3165 7531 (Singapore)
Toll Free +60 3 3099 4412 (Malaysia)
orders.singapore@partridgepublishing.com

www.partridgepublishing.com/singapore

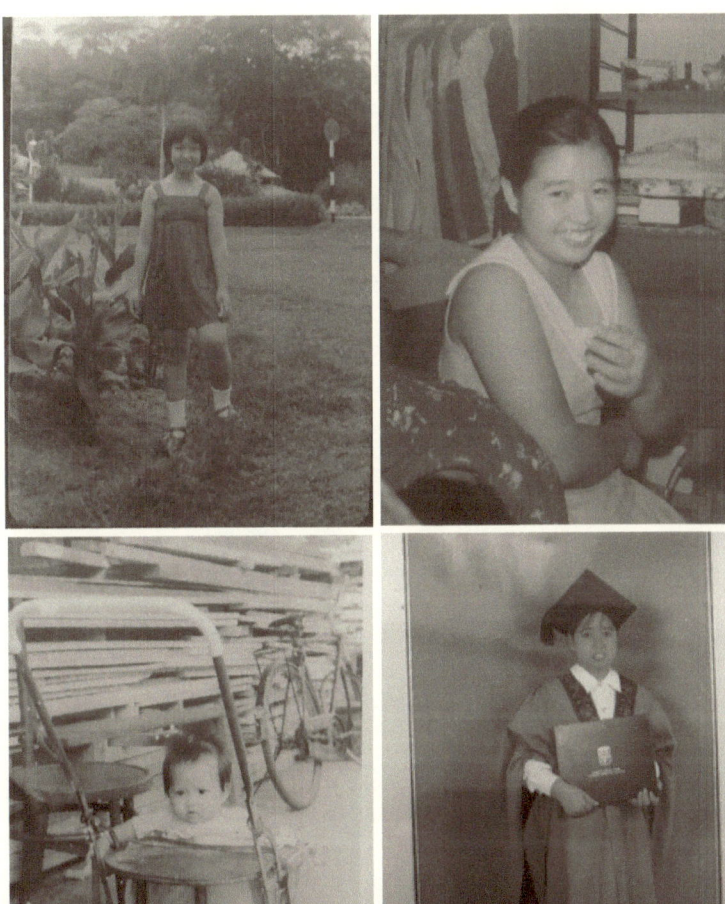

1

I struck lottery at the age of thirty-two—I was diagnosed with a brain tumour. After studying the CT scan, the GP had slowly revealed the news to me and my mother who had accompanied me to the hospital. I was thinking, *What, brain tumour?* It was so rare, you heard of people getting it, and I couldn't be the unlucky one. The doctor continued by saying that the brain tumour must be removed as soon as possible because it was so huge that the growth was pushing the brain to one side and pressing on the nerve, which explained the cause of pain and discomfort I felt for several years. Meanwhile, he mentioned that the hospital doesn't have the expertise or facilities to handle such surgery. He gave us a neurosurgeon's contacts and said that I should consult the neurosurgeon immediately. Instead of going immediately, my mother and I went home to let the grave news sink in. I couldn't clearly think after we left the doctor's room that I tried to exit from the parking at the entry point!

Once inside the car, Mom was full of questions, and it continued all the way home. 'Will everything be fine after the surgery? How long have you had those headaches? What caused the brain to have a growth? Is it something bad or just growth?' I provided the same answer to all the questions, which is 'I don't know'.

At home, I called to make an appointment with the neurosurgeon. The neurosurgeon could see me later in the afternoon.

We ate lunch in total silence. After leaving the GP's room, I have been imagining only one scenario: A surgery will be called for, then everything would be fine again, and life would be back to normal in no time; provided, of course, the tumour is not cancerous.

In the neurosurgeon's room, he studied the CT scan and then demanded a brain MRI. It had seemed like ages for the MRI result to be out. Finally, Mom and I were called into the neurosurgeon's room, we sat and waited anxiously for whatever he was going to tell us. Then he informed us that the tumour must be removed immediately via a brain surgery. He added that the risk of not removing the tumour is greater than the surgery itself because of the risk of the tumour bursting inside the brain. And if that were to happened, nothing could be done to save my life.

With the grave information in mind, we went home. Later in the evening, Mom relayed the news to my siblings who don't live in the family home.

The next day one of my sisters and her husband accompanied my mother and I to seek second opinion from another neurosurgeon, Dr Lee. After listening to our findings and studying the earlier MRI, Dr Lee ordered yet another brain MRI. It took like forever to see him about the MRI results because there were many people in the waiting area. At last, my name was called, and all four of us filed into the room. Dr Lee put up the film on a light box and explained. His explanation was about the same as the previous neurosurgeon, except that he had extra information to share. Dr Lee informed us that the tumour was like a ball measuring 3.5 cm in diametre. To our relief, he said that the growth is not cancerous, and he has removed such tumours in many patients in his more than twenty years' career as neurosurgeon. When we enquired, he said the success rate of the surgery is over 90 per cent. Dr Lee explained that before the brain surgery, he would carry out a procedure to ascertain whether there is any blockage in the brain, and if there was blockage, he would have to pull certain nerve from the leg to rectify the condition. He added that if we so decided, the brain surgery could be arranged on coming Friday; in that case, I would have to be admitted on Thursday for pre-surgery preparations. My mother and I have confidence in Dr Lee and the hospital he operated his clinic in, so we decided there and then that Dr Lee would be the neurosurgeon who would carry out the brain surgery on me. After going through all the necessary paperwork with Dr Lee's personal assistant, we were the last to leave his clinic long after normal operating hours.

Given that it was Tuesday, and I have to be admitted on Thursday, I was left with one day to arrange the necessary. So the next day was frantic for me. There were so much to handover in the office because we were in the final stage of planning a new store opening. Therefore, all seemed so sudden and rushed to say the least, applying medical leave, getting HR to prepare the relevant documentation in a day, cancelling meetings, explaining to the management, colleagues, and suppliers about my anticipated absence. All these left me with no time to find out more about brain tumours and the pending surgery and to tell my friends.

The saying 'ignorance is bliss' turned out to be true for me. Because of my lack of knowledge about brain surgeries and its possible aftermath, I have no fear and entered the operation theatre with a positive mind.

On 20 November 1998, I was wheeled into the operation theatre at 3:00 p.m. for craniotomy, a brain surgery that involved opening of the skull, four days after I was diagnosed with a brain tumour.

2

I used to have bouts of headache for several years. When it attacked, I became very moody. Thinking it might be caused by lack of sleep or the weather, I popped painkillers for quick relief. The headache would usually go off in an hour or two. I did the same in university and into my working life. What I did not realise was the painkillers had lost its effectiveness. I was feeling the pain for more and more hours. Sometimes I would be awakened in the middle of sleep by that sudden attack, and I have to call in sick the next day. GPs did not suspect anything amiss; they said the headache might be caused by migraine.

One afternoon in 1997, I felt something wobbled for a few seconds in my brain after I laughed vigorously. Not suspecting anything sinister, I did not pursue further.

During our last holiday to Yunnan, China, in March 1998, my holiday mood was badly disrupted by a lingering headache throughout the trip.

I couldn't sleep or eat well throughout the trip; I attributed the cause to be lack of sleeping time and the sudden changed in temperature as it was freezing cold in that part of China at that time. While we were travelling by train at night to Gui Yang, which means 'the sun is very expensive', the temperature was below-zero centigrade. I couldn't sleep on the train because of the lingering discomfort in my head, and it was very noisy. I think the noise was a result of train wheels grinding the track.

Sometime in the middle of the night, I felt a sudden nausea as I was going to the bathroom and vomited halfway to the washroom, much to the dismay of a lady attendant who reprimanded my mother and me. After we returned home, the headaches still occurred occasionally but with less intensity, and I did not look much into it.

In May 1998, my friends and I went to Club Med Cherating for a weekend. Even though the club served sumptuous food daily, it seemed I couldn't keep food down and vomited after every heavy meal. After vomiting, I would feel so lethargic and sleepy.

One Sunday in November 1998, after washing the car, a terrible headache was suddenly upon me. I took to sleep thinking I would feel better after some sleep, but I woke up feeling even worse, followed by a terrible vomiting spell 'til nothing came out but bile.

My mother was so alarmed that she insisted that I go for a thorough checkup. The next day, after listening to the story about headaches, the physician ordered a brain CT scan.

3

I lied very still and opened my eyes while trying to adjust to the surroundings; it was a dimly lit room. At the distance, a man was constantly coughing, a nurse was sitting in front of my bed, and I heard beeping sounds coming from a monitor beside the bed and realised that my head and hand were attached to various wires. I was feeling very thirsty and wanted some water, but it was impossible to call out to because of the oxygen mask over my face.

When I tried to move my limbs, to my horror, only the left hand was agreeable; the others refused to budge. I was literally three limbs down.

My mind was like asking, *What is happening?* I did not expect the result of the surgery to turn out this way. What would happen to me in the future? What about job? What about Mother? What about my plans and ambitions?

With my imagination running wild, I have so many questions, but nobody was around to answer them. I waited many hours before the nurses turned on the lights. Then Dr Lee came and checked on me. He explained to me that I was in ICU and that the surgery was a success. I gathered from Mom that the surgery lasted seven to eight hours, and everybody was waiting outside the operation theatre: Aunt Winnie, my sisters, and some of my friends. Dr Lee later informed my mother that I could be transferred out from ICU to a normal room in the afternoon.

For more than two weeks, I was totally bedridden and had to live with double vision. Speech required such great attempts, and it mostly came out in broken sentences. Totally bald and with a 270-degree scar on top of my head, my internal radiator also gone haywire. I would feel very warm when the room was already freezing cold. I couldn't turn my body, and even though the nurse came and turned my body, I couldn't sleep at night. However, I would be fast asleep when the nurses came to make the bed early in the morning. Besides that, my speech was slow, and I had double vision. Reasonably, I looked gloomy and down and would keep to myself the whole day. Dr Lee did explain that the mobility, speech, and eyesight issues I faced were temporary. Those were side effects. The nerves were disturbed when he was trying to excavate the tumour, and I would recover gradually. Nonetheless, I was thankful that my memory remained intact.

Throughout the two weeks, my condition caused me much anxiety and worry, not knowing whether I would fully recover to the way I was before the brain surgery. All kinds of doubts and uncertainty about the future entered my fragile mind. Every day the physiotherapist had to come in in order to administer treatment on me. After the physiotherapist left, my mother, who was accompanying me in hospital, would take over the role of physiotherapist. Other family members who came visiting also took turns to work as physiotherapist on me. By the end of the second week, to my relief and my family members', I had regained a fully-functioning left leg. Meanwhile, the right leg and hand movement showed improvement the following days. I was able to get out of bed and go to the Physiotherapy Department on the third week. According to the medical staff, it was a big achievement, but I was too occupied by present difficulties and worries to start celebrating this minor accomplishment. I was discharged at the end of third week to continue recuperation at home. Before discharge, I did check with the neurosurgeon what were the chances of a recurrence; his answer: 13 per cent. I found out later I had fallen into this percentage. Talk about unlucky numbers.

Four days after returning home, I was rushed to hospital again caused by a blood disorder; the red blood cells kept breaking, causing the hemoglobin and platelets level to drop to a dangerous level. This time the hematologist and nurses rallied around me. For more than a week, his attempt to determine the cause was unsuccessful. I was given blood infusion daily, but the hemoglobin level was unsatisfactory. As a last resort, the hematologist did a bone marrow biopsy for me. Miraculously, a day later, the red blood cells stopped breaking, and that day happened to be Christmas Eve 1998, and I was discharged for a second time after ten days.

Five months later, I returned to work, even though I still walked with a slight limb caused by the weakness of my right leg. My right ankle was not as flexible as before. My coordination and speech never got back to where they were before the brain surgery. On weekdays, I drove 50 km to the office where I was working as a buyer in a retail chain.

4

I remained an obedient patient, took medications on time, and went for doctors' appointment as scheduled. In order to regain my strength and improve balancing skill, I joined a gym with a swimming pool. I would go to the gym or pool every day after work. I underwent MRI every year.

The second annual MRI result showed no midline shift. However, the neurosurgeon detected a residual. He suggested that I get rid of the residual before it caused further neurological damage. Because the residual was very near to the aorta, invasive surgery was not an option.

The neurosurgeon recommended stereo static radio surgery (characterised by an intense beam targeted at the abnormal tissue while sparing normal tissue surrounding the affected area), which is also called gamma knife or laser. The neurosurgeon further explained that under this method, the surgery did not have to be invasive and the surrounding tissues would be spared any damage.

Therefore, in December 2000, I underwent the so-called SRS surgery. The preparation time by the medical team was much more than the actual surgery itself. The neurosurgeon literally screwed a robotic-looking helmet onto my head to prevent the head from moving during the procedure.

Once inside the operation theatre, a technician put a blindfold on me.

A few more personnel went to check again before I was left alone on a very cold table. The beam had to be applied a few times, each time at different angle; therefore, my head had to be shifted a few times.

Accuracy was highly important, and so were the mappings and calculations. The whole procedure took no more than two hours. I returned home the same day.

On June 2001, I was having lunch with colleagues when I felt a weird sensation rising from my right foot. The next moment, my whole body was in violent convulsion. The table, which I was holding, was shaking so hard as if in an earthquake. I lost consciousness in the process. After I came to, I spoke in a language foreign to my colleagues. Colleagues rushed me to the hospital. After, I was mentally awake but dazed. I felt so weak that I could barely walk. As I have called up earlier, the neurosurgeon was expecting me; he later explained that what I had been through just now was a type of seizure caused by epilepsy, very common in people with brain injuries; it was probably caused by a swelling or lesion in the brain. Whatever it was, I had to be admitted for observation. The onset of epilepsy affected the functionality of muscles on the right side of my body and right leg.

Overnight I found all the affected muscle groups weakened. I couldn't walk independently. I have lost natural balancing skill, and I have lost the ability to walk, which have come naturally since I was a toddler. Epilepsy also left me with immobile toes and ankle and coordination problems. The next day, after overnight observation, I was discharged with anticonvulsant drugs, which the neurosurgeon had prescribed, a drug which I would have to take for the rest of my life. The neurosurgeon recommended physiotherapy as treatment. When I asked, Dr Lee mentioned that I would not be able to walk or dance without assistance again.

When relevant drugs and initial physiotherapy didn't produce the results I was expecting, my hopes began to have doubts. As days turned into weeks, weeks turned into months and then years, I realised we were hoping against hope for a speedy recovery so life can go back as it was, but in my case, it seems there is no turning back the clock. Something already took shape in my mind even as we were seeking alternative treatment, traditional medicine both Chinese and Malay. We even visited various temples to seek for divine help, Christians chanted and prayed for me, but all failed to restore my physical ability and subsequently my soul. Fear, anxiety, worry, and negativities all got to me, and I forget how to smile, how to laugh, and how to be happy. To make matters worse, my weight jumped to 79 kg because of the steroids I was taking to control swelling of the brain. I became quiet, very quiet, too quiet. It didn't help when there was an incident where I fell face down. The impact of my weight caused the upper row of my front teeth to knock against the floor, which was the reason why I am wearing front upper row dentures now. If the diagnosis of brain tumour jolted me to the core, this disability totally floored me. I felt helpless, insecure, and not in control over everything even my own body. I was not able to go to work anymore and was officially medical boarded out in September 2001. This meant I officially stopped work after working for less than ten years. I felt miserable and restless every day, besides feeling cumbersome, burdensome, and a great inconvenience to others.

The emotional turmoil of watching the whole world crashing down on me was too much to bear; my social circle shrunk as I slipped into my own shell. Later signs of depression appeared when I started feeling emotional upheavals, having mood swing, and suffering from insomnia before having suicidal thoughts. I would wake in the middle of the night and cried myself to sleep. Luckily, it wasn't easy to end one's life when one was down and out. Furthermore, just the imagination of how sad my mother would be if her daughter should die before her was enough to stop me from committing the foolish act. I spent six years living like some hibernating creature. My brain couldn't perform any kind of multitasking. For example, I couldn't walk and think or talk at the same time. If I did those, I would certainly lose my balance. I wasn't interested in doing any exercise. I remained in the room most of the time. I needed assistance in going to the dining area or bathroom. I spent most days watching TV. Sometimes my mind was hijacked by the thinking that as an economics degree holder, I should do more instead of wasting my life away this way. So I read newspapers—the main paper, the business section, and the recruitment section—*Readers' Digest*, *National Geographic*, *Business Week*, etc. I was captivated by the thought that I should know about the current affairs and market situation and current developments well. I also screened the recruitment section every day, hoping to rejoin the workforce one day. I didn't realise that what I was thinking was unrealistic and unpractical. I was putting unnecessary pressure and stress on myself to the extent of hampering my recovery. There were many dark days as I struggled with self-denial and depression before I finally came to terms with the fact that I may have to live with what the doctors termed as progressive paralysis of the right side of the body.

One day, as I was watching TV, I am not sure what triggered me, perhaps an advertisement, a scene from a drama, or whatsoever. A fresh perspective began entering my mind. I realise that there was nothing I could do to change my immediate situation. Faced with the prospect of having to live with paralysis, the future looked gloomy. More than ever, it was a blow to see Mother taking care of me when I should be the one taking care of her and providing her with a comfortable life. Moreover, I did not want to become a wasted resource and another burden to society. Therefore, with the unrelenting encouragement and support of my family, I started physiotherapy again. In my mind, I was thinking it would be for my own good, if I could get stronger, and it wasn't fair to my mother as the primary carer. If I could get stronger and more independent after working on physiotherapy, it would make my mother's job easier. At the beginning, we changed the arrangement of stuff at home as much as possible so that they are accessible to me. Because of my immobility at the time, it was very inconvenient for me to travel. Therefore, I began physiotherapy at home. Deep inside, I was still hoping to shed the person with disability tag. I waited six years before registering as a disabled person with the state Welfare Department. From then on, I embarked on a vigorous rehabilitation program, which included physiotherapy and hydrotherapy in the hospital twice weekly and home physiotherapy. After months of diligent physiotherapy, I managed to slow down the progress of the paralysis and regained some muscle strength.

Rehabilitation is a hard, tedious, and long journey. I fell many times, picked myself up as many, and cried even more. I ended up with pain and bruises, but I was determined to continue. Eventually, my efforts of struggles, sweats, and tears did not go to waste. Positive results gradually, however stealthily, became obvious. My weight gone down, and my overall movement became easier as muscles began to build up.

Before physiotherapy, I needed a wheelchair for any kind of travelling, but after physiotherapy, I was able to use the walker for short distances. Throughout the years, I gained numerous scars, particularly on my knees and shoulders. I have a hairline fracture in my right shoulder while other bruises healed without leaving scars like fingers, thumbs, elbows, forearms, and buttocks. Usually, I tried my best to protect my head from knocking against something whenever I fall.

As if the medical issues concerning my physical condition were not bad enough, I was to enter the operation theatre once again for another medical condition. At some point before the brain tumour diagnosis, my biological cycle was disrupted without clear reason. Before the brain surgery, I had no menses for quite a couple of months, and then immediately after the surgery, menses commenced. It was a routine monthly thing until it stopped completely a few months later; I had thought it was caused by early menopause. Then the menses reappeared with a flurry after six years.

I suspected something was not right. After various tests returned negative results, the gynecologist I consulted suggested that I have a biopsy done on my uterus. As expected, the biopsy result pointed to abnormal activities in the uterus. After some medication, we did two more biopsies within one and a half years; the results were the same with the first one. If the condition were to continue, I ran the risk of developing cancer of the uterus, fallopian tubes, or ovaries. After contemplating the pros and cons and against the potential risk, I decided to have all three removed on 3 July 2012.

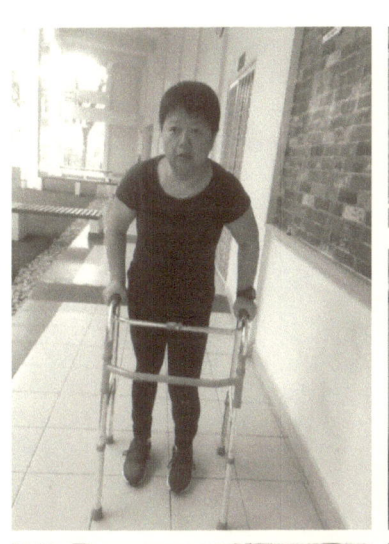
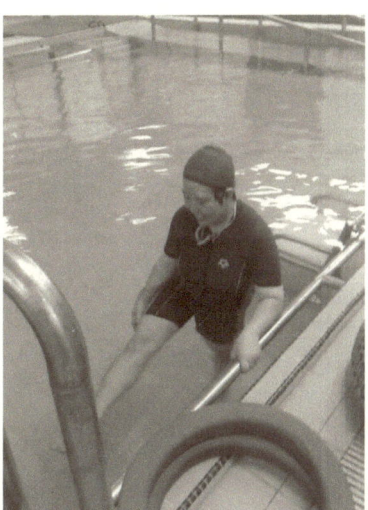
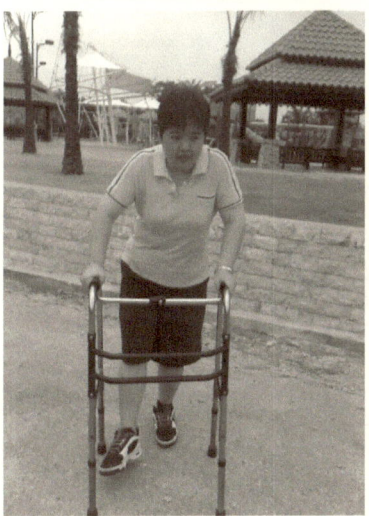
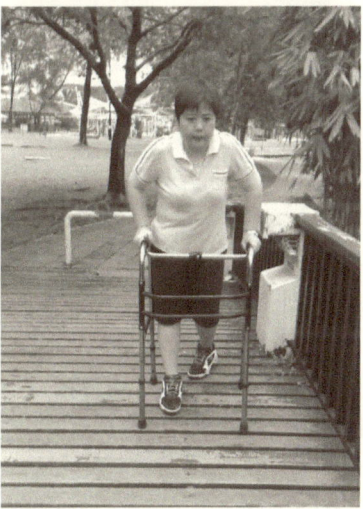

5

As a kid, I was the studious one among eight siblings.
I am the seventh child. My paternal grandmother,
my parents, and my two brothers and five sisters live
in a house made of solid wood. Initially, there were
three rooms in the house. My grandmother shared
a room with four of my sisters, my parents share a
room with me and my younger sister, and my two
brothers occupied one room. It is a nice house, the
bedrooms are big, the living room is spacious, and
there are areas for planting both in front and behind

the house. Over time we renovated the house into four rooms and then five rooms with spacious dining area and kitchen. It's a nice house, except for the address. The house is on a squatter area, surrounded by terrace houses, shop lots, condominiums. All amenities easily accessible from our location. At present, all my siblings are married, and they have their own houses. Our family house has more than enough rooms and sparsely occupied. I have turned one of the rooms into a mini gym to accommodate my stationary bike, treadmill, gym ball, dumbbells, a bench, and some bands and weights. The domestic helper has a room to herself. My brother and his wife occupied one room, while their children has another room.

My mother and I shared a room since my father passed away more than thirty years ago.

I have witnessed three deaths of my loved ones. My grandmother passed away because of throat cancer when I was twelve. Six months prior to her death, she was literally starved to death. Neither food nor drink, nothing, could pass through her esophagus. My father died of cardiac arrest when I was twenty-one. It was very sudden. Then just about sixteen months ago, dear aunt Winnie breathed her last because of final-stage sarcoma cancer in the lung. For three months, I witnessed her once strong body devoured by the deadly disease.

My mother is ninety going ninety-one. I am so thankful she can still do the things she enjoys, like cooking and making delicacies. It is my responsibility to keep track on her medical appointments, which involves orthopaedic, chiropractor, physiotherapist, and other routine checkups in the hospitals. I am also attentive on her food intake, and I make sure the supply of her medicine and supplement is sufficient. I am lucky to have the support of my siblings, in-laws, and nieces whenever I need help. After my father passed away, my mother struggled to hold the family together. At that time, I got an offer to further my studies in a local university. My mother encouraged me to accept the offer, and I did. I struggled financially throughout the four years in the university. After graduation, I worked with a retail company. I started in the operations department before I was transferred to the merchandising department. It was my first job, and it turned out to be my last before I was medically boarded out. During the nine years I was working, I took my mother for year-end holidays in Australia, on a cruise, in Shanghai, Bangkok, Pattaya, and Southern China.

At ninety, my mother loves festive gatherings and cooks for her brood of eight children, seven in-laws, twenty-two grandchildren, and seventeen great-grandchildren. I am so proud of my mother, and I pray that she will continue to be healthy and happy for many years to come.

6

Appointments with neurosurgeons and annual MRI have become my routine since the brain surgery. Between 2006 and 2011, the MRI showed no growth or enlargement of the scarred tissue. Then the break came in 2013, when the MRI did not pick up any residuals, scarred tissues, or lesion in the brain, which means my brain is clear of anything affecting the nerves. At last, I heard the news I had been waiting for since the fateful day on 1 June 2001. Upon hearing this piece of news, my sense of accomplishment and confidence grew a few knots, and my hope of moving around using less assistance increased by leaps and bounds. By then, I have gained much muscle strength, and the light at other end of the tunnel suddenly shone ever brighter. Sometime after knowing about the good news, I felt my weight distribution and overall balancing improved. Realising I still have a long way to go, I continued with physiotherapy to improve on flexibility, emphasising on quality of the voluntary movements of joints as well as gait.

Despite my condition, I possessed the desire in me to improve myself or learn or improved on things I am interested in if the opportunity arises. I have been a swimmer prior to the disability, and I occasionally swam in the hydrotherapy pool after finishing physiotherapy routine, but only if the physiotherapist gave permission for me to do so. However, hydrotherapy pools were not meant for swimming. It measures only 3 m x 2.5 m.

When a friend informed me about an NGO organising a diving, whereby they would bring people with disabilities on diving trips and they would be conducting swimming classes in a swimming pool, I jumped on the opportunity immediately and promptly registered as a participant. Swimming classes took place for two hours every Sunday morning, three months prior to the diving trip. During those three months, two of my nieces drove me to the swimming pool, waited for me to complete my classes, took me to lunch before sending me home again.

Two weeks before the trip, we held two sessions, one for snorkeling practice and another for diving.

The date we were waiting for had arrived, and we were all ready for the trip, and it was to be a five-day, four-night trip to Tioman Island.

The organiser's aim was to make it to the Malaysia Book of Records by getting the most disabled people to dive for thirty minutes at the depth of twenty feet below sea level.

Our contingent consisted of thirty-one persons with disabilities, sixty-three volunteers, and twenty dive instructors who would be waiting on the island for our arrival. On 21 August 2014, we gathered at Setia Walk, Puchong, at 10:00 p.m. As all participants slowly trickled in, the whole waiting area was like the waiting area in the airport. A table was set up as a temporary checking-in counter. After all the wheelchairs, walking devices, and luggage were tagged according to four colours, the participants were then separated into groups of six. Each group consisted of two disabled persons and four volunteers; we were told to identify our group members in order to be able to seek out one another when we needed help.

When it came to boarding the bus, luggage and wheelchairs of the same colour tags were loaded into a bus's luggage compartment. For those who could stand and walk, the volunteers supported them all the way 'til they were safely seated. For those who could not stand, the volunteers would carry them to their seats. The same process was carried out when people with disabilities were getting down from the buses. Finally, we set off in four buses at midnight. During the journey, we stopped twice for supper and toilet breaks.

We arrived at Tanjung Gemok, Mersing, at about 7:00 a.m.; we had breakfast in one of the old coffee shops. After breakfast, all wheelchair users were wheeled to the jetty nearby, and the buses sent our luggage to the jetty. We spent roughly three hours in the hall of the jetty because the first ferry service started at 11:30 a.m. During which time, our volunteers had enough time to sort out the luggage and some paperwork.

When the ferry arrived, our volunteers had to transfer the luggage to the ferry first, then came the transferring of wheelchair users. The process of embarking the ferry was similar to boarding the bus, except that transferring to the ferry was more dangerous and challenging because of more stone steps leading to the ferry. Somehow our enthusiastic volunteers managed to get all disabled people onboard safely.

The ride in ferry took about two and a half hours. During which, I found out that there are a few kampongs in Tioman Island because the ferry made two to three stops for passengers to embark and disembark. Finally, we reached our destination and the ferry's final stop Kampung Salang.

Once there, the diving instructors from a local dive centre and their staff were on hand to greet us. We headed for lunch while they sort out the luggage. After lunch, we were given our room keys. When we came back for our luggage, we were assigned life jackets and snorkeling masks and told to return on the last day of the trip. The room arrangements were so that we had two or three volunteers sharing a room with a disabled person. I later gathered that most of the volunteers are certified divers of various levels. During each snorkeling and diving sessions, at least two volunteers would be supporting each disabled participant. Before going on the trip, I was somehow worried about the activities the organiser had planned. I was afraid that volunteers might not be able to see and find me if I went missing. Therefore, I had bought myself a swimsuit in a very bright colour (glows-in-the-dark yellow).

We had a few snorkeling sessions the following day. In the morning, we rode speedboats to a snorkeling site, and later, at lunch, we went to another snorkeling site. With the sea surrounding us, the rides on speedboat were windy and exhilarating.

It reminded me of the times my friends and I rode on jet skis. The memory and the moment brought tears to my eyes. We managed to see the life in the underwater world with plenty of colourful fishes and corals besides other flora and fauna. After snorkeling in the sea, we went back to our rooms for some rest before we went snorkeling again in the evening, this time near the beach.

Our most anticipated activity fell on the fourth day—dive by person with disabilities. We gathered for briefing at 9:00 a.m. In order to avoid taking unnecessary risk, the organiser and diving instructors placed safety on top of everything else. They had planned five people with disabilities to dive at each time; hence, people with disabilities were divided into six groups.

Each person would have one dive instructor dive with him/her supported by a dive master. Our diving expedition would take thirty minutes; during which time, we would have the rare opportunity for our pictures taken under the sea by a photographer. During the briefing, I was so excited and moved that I became teary-eyed. I got emotional because after I became disabled, I have never imagined involving myself in challenging sports activities, let alone diving. It sounded so surreal that after all these years, I still have the opportunity to make it happen. During the dive, I felt total freedom in the sea; no barriers, no limitation, no structural or architectural obstacles, and certainly, nobody was staring. I felt zero gravity, floating among fishes, corals, and other fauna and flora of the marine world. For disabled participants, this opportunity to dive might well be the chance of a lifetime for them. This is mainly because friends and relatives might consider diving too dangerous; furthermore, this activity required group effort to ensure its success because the journey to a diving paradise would not be easy, especially with the participation of people with disabilities.

I am very grateful to all the volunteers and diving instructors. The volunteers had accompanied us all the way throughout the trip, on land and in sea. Without them, this experience of a lifetime would not be possible.

Diving was such an adventurous activity that I joined the event for the following four consecutive years. Can you imagine the feeling of being surrounded by school of fishes of all colours and sizes while swimming at sea? I would say it was the most exciting, fantastic, and dreamlike feeling with all the fishes seemingly swimming together with you. It was both exciting and fascinating that when your hand held out some bread, all the fishes swooped by together, and each tried to take a bite on it. Besides, when you look down, not far away from your feet, you could see a lot of beautiful corals and various sea-grown mushrooms, and there were sea cucumbers sitting very still in between these. That much can be said from my recent snorkeling experience. However, scuba diving is a very different story.

In scuba diving, we have to wear all the necessary gears and the heavy-looking oxygen tanks. Although some of the things seen during diving was the same in snorkeling, as you go deeper under the sea, more marine life could be discovered, and if you were lucky, you would see boxfish or nemo fish, turtles, little sharks, and other not-so-common fishes. In addition, we actually saw a post box under the sea! The feeling of diving was one of total peace and freedom; there were no obstacles or any type of discrimination. I felt like an astronaut circulating space.

We dived in Redang Island in 2015; in Mabul, Sabah, in 2016; and in Perhentian Islands in 2017 and 2018. As the years progressed, people with disabilities were given more dives in each event, from one dive throughout the trip in Tioman Island in 2014 to four dives in Perhentian Islands in 2018.

After the diving trips, I continued practicing swimming consistently. I swim for two hours every weekend. Initially, the right side of my body kept sinking, and I could not manage 6 m at a time, but this changed gradually as I could swim 12 m and then 36 m and 48 m. After practicing for about a year, I did not even realise when my body started to be in balance while swimming. However, because I am living with epilepsy, I just could not summon enough courage to swim the full 50 m length, even though my epilepsy was very well controlled. I must have someone to accompany me every time before I swim the full length of the pool. Finally, I paid a coach to teach me some self-rescue techniques and train me to swim in laps. After four lessons, I was confident enough to swim the full 50 m and then 100 m, followed by 200 m, 300 m, 400 m, and so on. After the first diving experience, getting a diving certificate sounded far more tempting; the only thing that was holding me back was the word 'epilepsy'.

As my epilepsy was well controlled and chances of me suffering a seizure were almost zero, in 2016, doctors in Neurosurgery Department suggested that I further reduce my dosage of anticonvulsant drugs. The positive signs had boosted my confidence, and I dared to dream of being certified as a scuba diver in the near future. And it was during the diving event in Mabul Island that I got my certification as a scuba diver. The trip to Sabah also created much memories in me and my fellow disability comrades because we conquered all three modes of transportation—land, air, and sea.

It was the diving trip in 2015 and 2016 when we had friends from China, Hong Kong, and Poland participate in the adventure. It was interesting to learn that they used to dive in lakes in Poland. Diving is a new experience for those from Hong Kong and China. These activities were an eye-opening experience to the various types of disabilities people are dealing with on a daily basis—just to name a few, there's spinal cord injury, amputation, polio, vision impairment, learning disabilities, muscular dystrophy, and arthritis—and they are living with various levels of severity. While some of these disabilities lead to people becoming wheelchair users, others end up using various mobility devices.

On 28 July 2016, sixty volunteers and twenty persons with disabilities took the 7:45 a.m. flights with two different airlines from Kuala Lumpur International Airport and arrived in Kota Kinabalu International Airport at about three hours later.

Our co-organiser in Sabah greeted our arrival warly. They had prepared several SUVs, vans, and two buses to ferry our group to the jetty. From the jetty, we took speedboats to Semporna Island. The dining hall of the dive centre served as our venue for dining, briefing, and socialising.

We were lucky, for the weather was good in the following two days. We went diving two times a day, in the morning and in the afternoon. It rained heavily on the evening of 30 July, and the wind was strong. The following morning, our morning dive had to be postponed to the afternoon because of strong wind and current. Even during the afternoon dive, the visibility was not good. On this trip, I learned how to perform back roll from the boat with diving gears on. I have seen people doing it on TV and videos and thought it was cool, and now I could do the same—fantastic.

We left Semporna Island after early breakfast on 1 August to catch the 9:00 a.m. flights. That morning, it was raining accompanied by mild wind and current. The boat ride to the jetty was bumpy, and then we took the prearranged buses to Kota Kinabalu, where we had lunch before heading to Kota Kinabalu International Airport. Again, our contingent boarded two separate aircrafts for Kuala Lumpur. I left Kota Kinabalu knowing I am now a certified scuba diver, and when I received the PADI diver card some three weeks later, I felt oddly happy and proud.

It was a horrifying when I noticed a dive site full of what looks like broken bones. All seemed whitewash after being dead for a long time. When I swam nearer and took a better look, my fears were allayed because what I thought were broken bones were actually demised corals.

The shrinking coral reef in local marine parks is caused by a harsh environment, overdevelopment, rubbish, and too much chemical like sun protection oil in the sea. Divers, snorkelers, unknowingly or accidentally, killed some corals. The consequence of climate change and global warming made it much more difficult to preserve the beauty of these nature's gifts to the ecosystem of marine life. Prior to the above experience, I was not aware of the danger posed by humans on coral reefs. I discovered such hideous site during one of the dives in Pulau Perhentian, during our diving trips on 20-23 July 2017. One of the highlights of the diving trip was coral conservation. Therefore, throughout these diving outings, divers were repeatedly reminded against contaminating the sea with rubbish, chemicals, touching or kicking the corals.

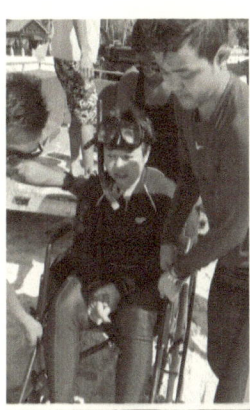
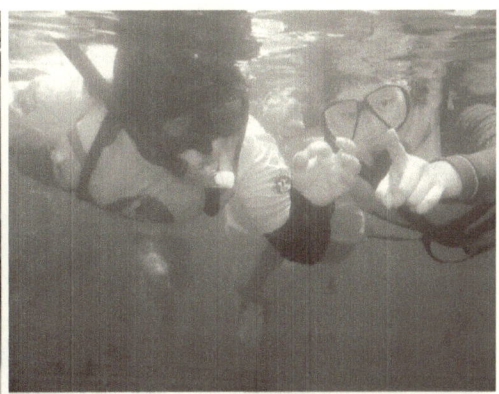
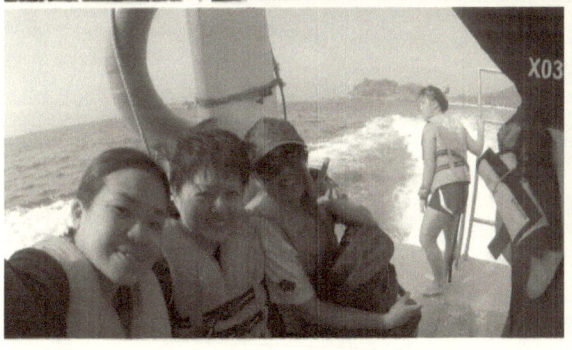
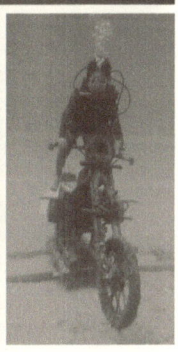

7

For several times a week, I take a morning walk around the neighbourhood. This exercise is always carried out in the presence of my helper. We set out with the necessary accessories: my walking frame, wrist protectors, and sports sandals.

We start by negotiating the drain and the cemented rough patch in front of my house. Then I need to use all my strength to haul myself up and balance my whole body on the road, which is on a higher level.

Holding on to the walker, I make a 90-degree turn in the direction we are heading. We begin our morning walk from that point. Throughout the walk, I have the opportunity to observe and meet various people who live in the neighbourhood.

There is this pleasant gentleman who enjoys walking his dog and always stops to greet me 'good morning.' He would enquire after my well-being and engage in a bit of small talk before cheerfully waving me off. Then there is this lovely couple in their late fifties who enjoy a brisk walk around the neighbourhood after walking their dogs.

Another familiar face is that of a kind lady in her seventies.

This spirited septuagenarian is full of encouragement and always has a nice word for everyone. She takes turns to visit her grandchildren who live in different parts of the city. But home to her is this humble dwelling where she has been living for the past fifty years.

Then there is this retired nurse in her sixties who lives alone. The nephew who used to live with her succumbed to brain tumour more than a year ago. This lady has even offered to massage my lower limbs to help improve blood circulation. Almost all of them asked similar questions when we met for the first time. The questions revolved around the events that led to my disability.

'What happened to you? Did you fall and injured your leg? Did you have a stroke?' they would ask.

'No, I am a brain tumour survivor. I had a growth in the brain,' was my standard reply.

'Oh dear. Did you have an operation? How long ago? How come the brain affects your leg?' they would enquire with concern.

'Yes, I underwent an operation about twenty-two years ago. Our brain has a lot of nerves. It's just liked a computer's CPU. If something goes haywire in the CPU, the computer will not function properly. Same thing here. If part of the brain has been damaged, then certain parts of the body will not work properly.'

Their next response: 'Are you still on medication? What did the doctor say? Will you recover?'

'Yes, I am on certain types of medication,' I explained. 'The doctor says something about scar tissue pressing on the nerves. Nobody can say for sure if I can recover to my pre-tumour condition, but the doctor said physical therapy would help, and here I am, working very hard at it.'

The answer to their last question brought regret to some faces, while others expressed relief and offered words of encouragement.

Some pointed out that I am lucky to come through with only my mobility affected; they have heard of patients who lost their sight, hearing, memory, and even their lives.

I remember one guy who responded in his own unique way: '*Aiyo*, if you cannot recover, you will spend the rest of your life with this disability.

So pitiful *lah*.'

At that moment, I thought to myself, *Do I look pathetic to him?*

His response painted a picture of how ignorant and insensitive some people can be at times. I started imagining how these people would cope with their life if they were in my shoes. Hide in their own shells, maybe?

We may have our physical limitations, but we try to overcome or work around them. For me, it is a constant process of trying, falling, picking up again, and adapting. Sooner or later, we will find ways to adapt to our circumstances. And the sooner we learn to live with ourselves, the better it is for us.

It isn't easy learning to live with a disability. There were times when the challenges seemed insurmountable. Trying to live with accessible facilities, or the lack of it, is a norm for the disabled community in Malaysia. Logistics is always an issue in any outing. Previously, before e-hailing vehicles come into play, I rely mostly on taxis for transport. Sad to say, some taxi drivers would not stop for me. Some pretended that they did not see me when I tried to wave down a taxi.

Then there are taxi drivers who take advantage of disabled passengers. They charge extra for boot usage despite a ruling from the Commercial Vehicle Licensing Board (LPKP) that there should be no extra charges under the new fare system.

Once, when I complained about the charges and tried to jot down the cabbie's particulars so that I could lodge a complaint with LPKP later, the driver ticked me off when he realised what I was trying to do.

Feeling vulnerable and afraid that I would be harmed, I alighted without taking the cab's particulars.

Like any other shopper, I enjoy retail therapy once in a while. I like to hang out at Suria KLCC because of its disabled-friendly facilities. But there's one thing that baffles me: The toilets for the disabled are always locked. I have to ask the cleaners to unlock the toilet each time I need to use it. However, not every cleaner has the key!

As all the cleaners are either Indonesians or Bangladeshis, they are not around between 12:45 p.m. and 2:45 p.m. on Fridays, as they are out for lunch or need to go to the mosque for prayers, so I avoid visiting this premier shopping mall on Fridays.

I also like to shop at AEON because it is well equipped with facilities for the disabled. Just like any abled-bodied person, the disabled enjoys the simple pleasures of life. We make the best of our circumstances and are thankful for the blessings that come our way. Many of the hurdles in our path are man-made. With a little more empathy from society, we hope to overcome barriers and push into new frontiers. Life has its share of challenges, whether we are able-bodied or disabled. Like they say, it is what we make of what we have that matters most.

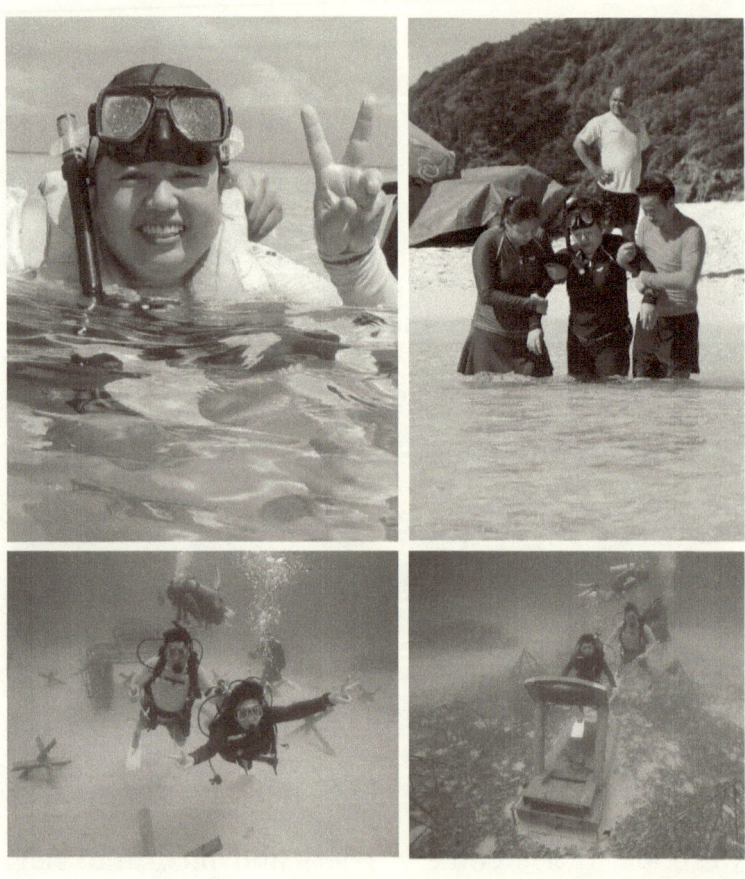

8

Physiotherapy, exercise, or workout, whatever you call it, became part of my daily routine. I go for walks two or three times a week on weekdays. I cycle or do indoor exercise on the days I don't go walking. Initially, I was worried that my physical condition will deteriorate if I stop exercising, like my limbs won't follow instructions. However, as time passes, the activities become a natural part of my life. This led to me looking for other forms of exercise; I have tried wheelchair tennis but found it too tough, then I heard and Googled about Pilates. In May 2017, I went for the assessment in a Pilates studio. When I arrived there in my wheelchair, I was dismayed to find that the studio was located on the first floor, and the walkway on the ground was covered with grass and gravel. A male staff helped me up to the studio. He huffed and puffed trying to maneouvre my wheelchair to a lift at the end of the building before finally getting to the studio. The studio was situated at the end of a row of link houses, which had been converted into business premises. The lift for wheelchair users was at the other end of the building. With all the grass, gravel, stoned path, curbs, and steps, how on earth did the developer expect a wheelchair user was going to get to the lift was beyond me. Because many shop lots were vacant, the accessible toilet was in an isolated spot with nobody around. When I complained about the inaccessibility of the studio to the staff, they informed me that they were moving to a new premise, which was under renovation. The new studio is right opposite the current studio, and it's going to be equipped with accessible facilities.

In March 2018, I went to the newly-renovated studio for another assessment, with the purpose to conduct a site survey in mind. The premises are a converted bungalow with a studio upstairs, and there is another one on the ground floor. There is an accessible washroom within the studio on the ground floor. At the main entrance, the surface is flat, and there is a ramp leading up to the studio. I have been going for my weekly Pilates session in this studio since then. In the first few sessions, I wasn't able to perform a lot of movements. I needed the instructor's assistance in positioning my right leg in the starting position. After every session, the instructor would give me 'homework' so that I could practice at home. Sometimes, after a tough session, I experienced muscle soreness and needed rest for two to three days. The instructors used to tell me that pain is good; that means the intended muscles are working. So far, I am satisfied with my progress. Imagine my sense of achievement when I managed to do plank a couple of months ago! And the instructors told me that I have become a star student in the centre!

I have always been interested in physical activities: swimming, diving, runs, fun rides, exercise, etc. I bought a motor attachment for my wheelchair so I could participate in fun rides. With the attachment, I am able to visit booths set up on grass surface at carnivals. Grass surfaces can be tricky to wheel or push a wheelchair. I am a tennis fan for both men and women players. I tried wheelchair tennis, but it was too difficult for me; I prefer watching tennis matches. I joined others in Kuala Lumpur Car Free Morning organised by Kuala Lumpur City Council on first and third Sundays of the month, from 7:00 a.m. to 9:00 a.m. If the weather permits, I would go for a ride in the parks. I don't enjoy travelling so much because if I spent so much in travelling, I prefer to appreciate the sightseeing and everything else from an eyelevel of at least 1.5 m or more instead of 1 m. Furthermore, there are other intangible baggage when travelling as a disabled person.

Fret not, I have found a way where one could enjoy the surroundings without limit—yes, the gravity-defying diving. This is an activity I may spend more time doing. Recently, I joined a weekly exercise session conducted by researchers at the University of Malaya Disability Sport Research Centre. These free sessions aim to encourage people with disabilities to be physically active by introducing various inclusive exercises.

It is very important to stay physically active to stay healthy. This is true particularly with people with disabilities. Because of our limited mobility, we tend to live quite sedentary lifestyles, which could lead to muscle wastage and result in reduced strength and osteoporosis, not to mention diseases like high blood pressure and diabetes.

I participated in The Catwalk of Malaysia 2018 held on 9 December. There were twelve of us in the Unique Star category, with seven being wheelchair users and five using various walking devices. I ended up winning first runner-up. Prizes included a certificate, a trophy, and RM500.

I drew plenty of positivity from the encouragement shown by the spectators, emcees, and judges.

9

Year 2020 is a crazy year. At the time of writing, there are nearly 60 million people infected with coronavirus and almost 1.4 million deaths worldwide, and the race to be number one in the world with the most people infected is scary. The world is in lockdown. After the first wave of coronavirus, countries are cautiously easing movement control rules while trying very hard to contain a second or third wave of the deadly and highly-infectious virus. People are advised to work from home, avoid crowds, and avoid close interaction with one another. Schools, colleges, and campuses are closed, and students are told to study online from home. With borders closed and planes grounded, many people are separated from their loved ones.

World economy is at rock bottom. Even big names are winding up their business. Layoffs and pay cuts are unavoidable in some companies that chose to continue running. The frontlines found themselves tired, separated from their loved ones, and laymen are suffering from pandemic fatigue. All these factors are contributing to people feeling under unrelenting stress and develop mental health issues subsequently. With all the negativities around, I think a little positivity will help. Hence, I decided to publish *Rising* in the midst of this pandemic.

If I could rise from something as scary as brain tumour, I think everybody has the ability to rise from whatever their circumstances might be, however difficult it might seem. Humans possess survival instinct.

My present state of health? I would say it is still a work in progress. Physically, I can't walk independently. I needed a walker to walk. When I walk, I have to be very focused so as not to lose my balance, especially when I want to turn. Any distraction—talking, thinking, analysing—would cause me to fall. My right toes cannot move voluntarily; my right ankle cannot move at all. I walk with a hyperextended right knee, and my right hip function is not up to par.

I can't write legibly. I have to take a nap in order to function well.

I can't sit too long for my joints won't do their job well if I did. Rushing make my nerves jump. That's why sometimes I use wheelchair for ease. When I am seated, I can do anything, and nobody can tell that I am a person with disability. I hope to continue improving and rising so that I would be able to live more independently. So I would continue keeping at all the exercise routine. Meanwhile, I am still exploring more reasons for my existence.

The last crowded event I attended in 2020 was during Chinese New Year in February. It was a charity event when once again I was given the opportunity to walk in cheongsam on stage. It was held just before COVID-19 was declared a pandemic. Some of my scheduled activities were disrupted; no swimming, no Pilates, no roaming in the parks, no shopping, no lunch appointments; just staying at home as much as possible.

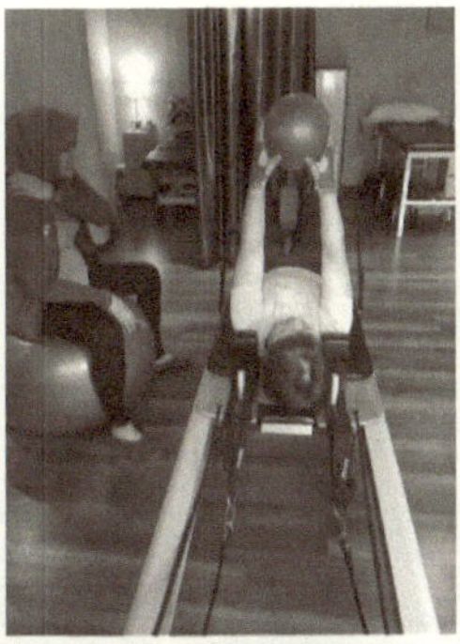

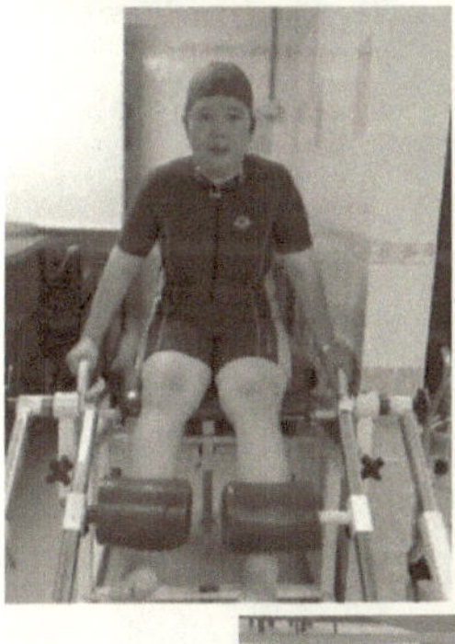

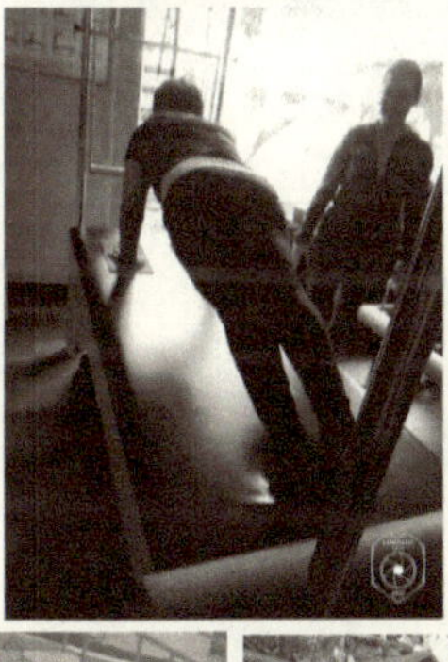

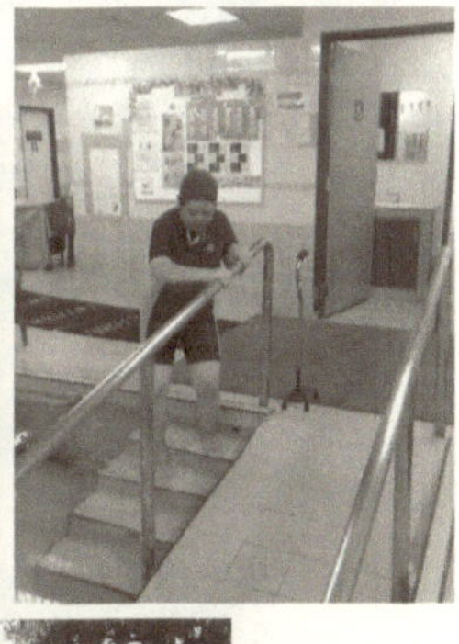

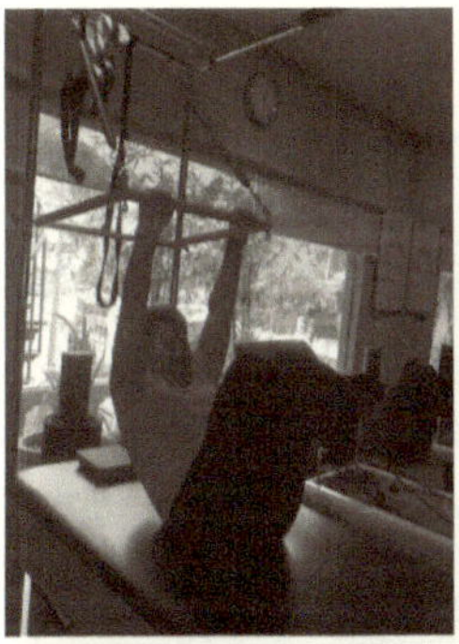

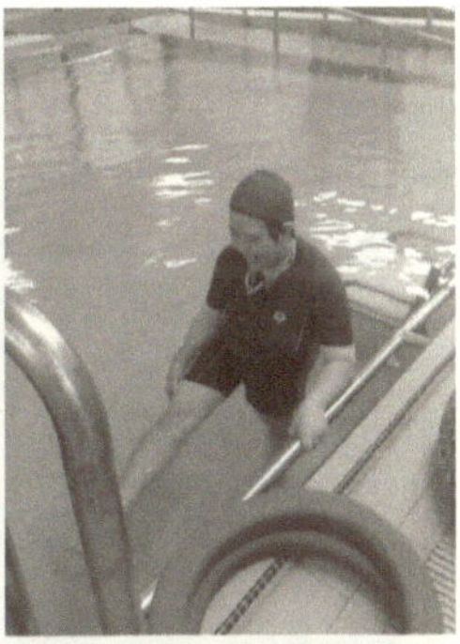

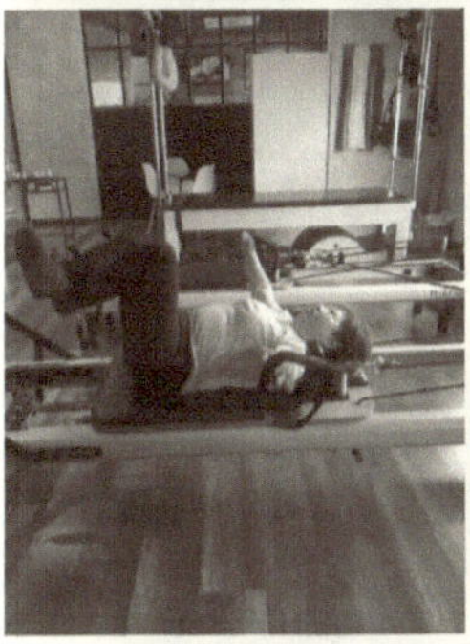

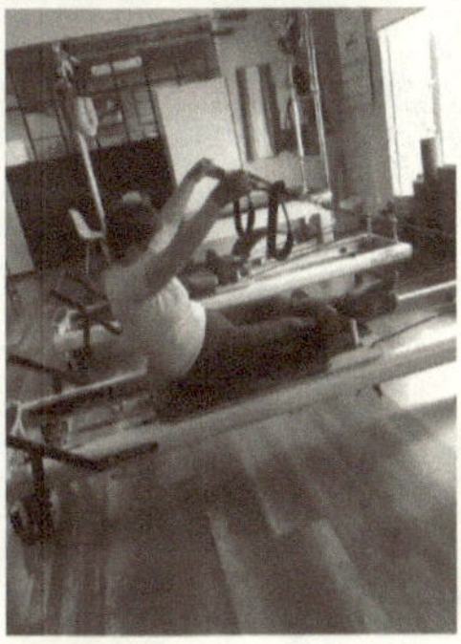

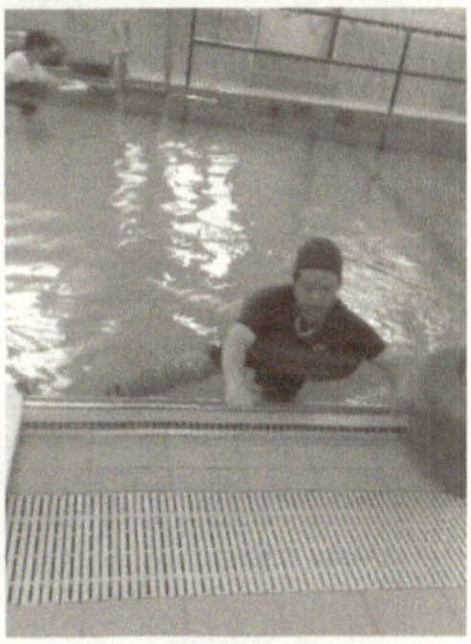

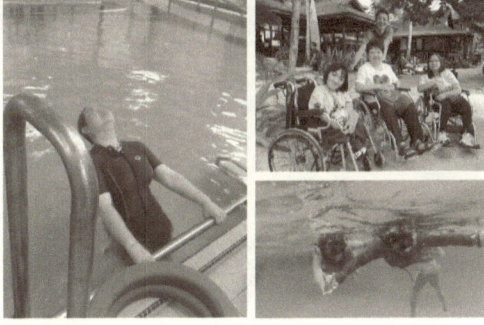

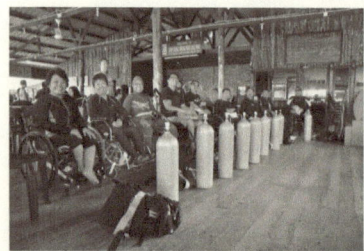
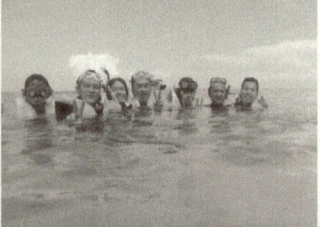
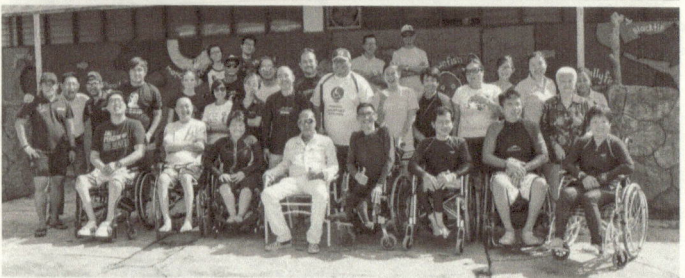
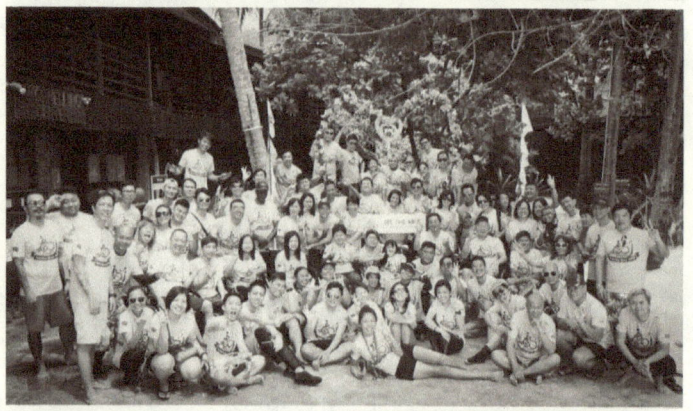
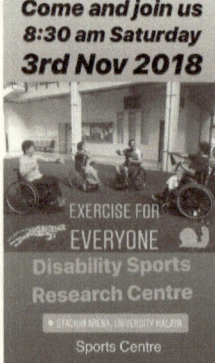

Come and join us
8:30 am Saturday
3rd Nov 2018

EXERCISE FOR
EVERYONE
Disability Sports
Research Centre
STADIUM ARENA, UNIVERSITY MALAYA
Sports Centre

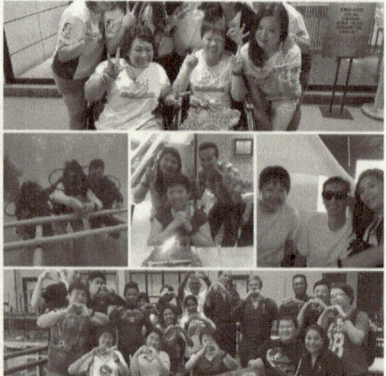

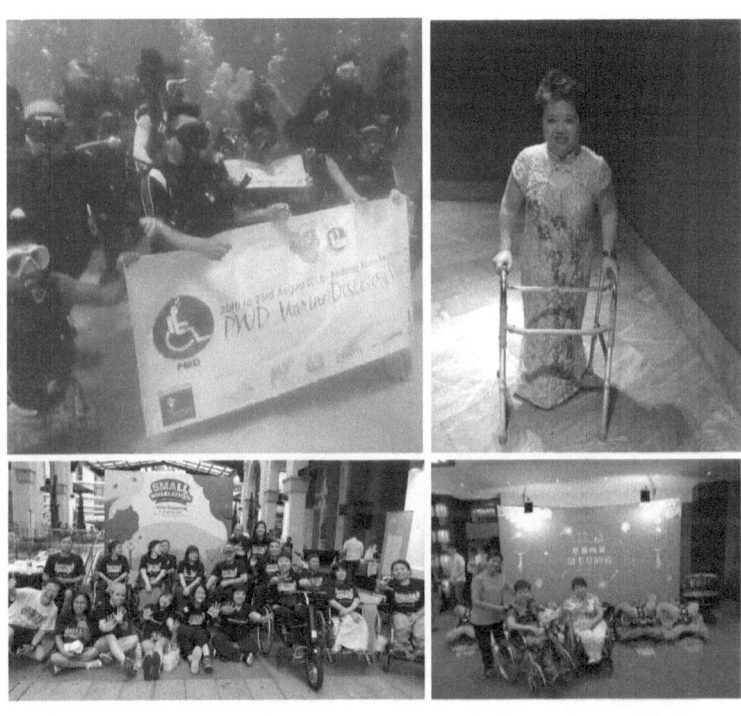